PAIN

FREE

AFTER

60

BY LORRAINE J-WILKES

Pain Free After Sixty

A Journey to Inner Healing
Tips and Guides for Pain
Management Without Costly
Medications

COPY RIGHT

Table of Contents

The Six Signs of Inflammation 1

Wellness Plan 2

Promise to Myself 3

Fruits good for Juicing & Eating 4

Vegetables for Juicing & Eating 5

Juicing Recipes 6

Acknowledgements

Thank you to my Lord and Savior Jesus

Christir for   Salvation.

In Memory of Mary Rose Jenkins, my dear

mother who fought hard for her health.

To My Husband Donnie Ray Wilkes. You

are my   ray of sunshine. Thank you for your

unfailing support.

To My Son Jeffery, thank you for believing

in the   vision and being my Brand Manager. This

book was your idea.

Thank you to all the support from my family

Introduction

I have dedicated my life to healthcare for over four decades. After serving the community for two decades, I developed more than 10,000 diets for geriatric clients. I also became an Executive Director in healthcare. Throughout my career, I have always maintained an active lifestyle and enjoyed promoting the benefits of good nutrition.

A Personal Promise to Achieve the Best in Life

Upon reaching the age of 60, I made a promise to myself to be the best version of me in various areas of life. These areas include health, wealth, love & relationships, finance, self-esteem, and personal development. However, I encountered a significant obstacle that challenged my promise. I was experiencing excruciating pain and inflammation in my knees, hips, back, and upper arms, which made it impossible to exercise and led to weight gain. Despite this, I only shared my struggle with a few close relatives and my husband. I felt vulnerable sharing it with others, even at work.

A Journey to Finding Relief from Pain

After seeking medical attention from multiple specialists without any positive results, I was left disappointed. As someone who has worked with doctors in healthcare for years, I even tried pharmaceuticals but experienced negative side effects. I eventually stopped taking the medication and tried alternative remedies like heating pads and creams, which would work for some time, but then the pain would return. It wasn't until I prayed that I realized the solution was closer than I thought. My husband, who is 70 years old, did not experience any of the issues that I was going through.

I watched my husband mix his healthy drinks day after day. I asked him what he was doing. "He said I am juicing for my health.: He gave me some of his drinks several times. I could not drink it because of the taste. He went to his doctor and received good reports. He was not taking any medications. I decided to do my research and find juice that would help and taste good to me. I began juicing. I worked in all of the areas that I needed improvement in my life. After getting my health under control. I knew other people were also suffering, and thus, my journey to help others. Join me as I continue my journey to being pain-free after 60 and taking care of the whole person.

It's amazing how a journey to finding relief from pain can lead to a new lifestyle and even a mission to help others. Juicing is just one example of how small changes in our daily routines can have a big impact on our health. Through research and experimentation, this journey led to a discovery of a variety of healthy and delicious juice recipes that not only provided relief from pain, but also improved overall wellbeing.

This journey to being pain-free after 60 is not just about physical health, but also about taking care of the whole person. It's about finding balance, nourishing the body with healthy foods and drinks, and taking care of the mind and spirit. Through this journey, the goal is to help others who may be experiencing similar pain and discomfort. Join us on this journey to transform living spaces and lives, one healthy choice at a time.

Chapter one

The 6 Signs of Inflammation

Have you ever heard of silent inflammation? Simply put – this harmful inflammation is the "mortal enemy" of your health. It can damage your heart and brain, throw your digestive system completely out of whack, make your joints stiff and achy, and even ruin the color and texture of your skin. It's irrefutable at this point – more and more scientific research is clearly showing that **silent inflammation is the common link** that fast-tracks aging and makes us look and feel old before our time. So, reducing silent inflammation throughout your body may be the **single most important thing** you can do on a daily basis to look and feel your best. As scientists begin to understand the body's complex systems better, a clearer picture of how every day, silent inflammation can impact your health is emerging. Here are six of the most common symptoms:

Memory Impairment:

Research has shown that when the brain is inflamed, memory formation and recall both suffer. Unfortunately, many people start to believe that scattered thoughts and trouble focusing are an inevitable part of aging—but they're not! Silent inflammation is likely the culprit.*

Cholesterol Imbalances:

A growing body of evidence has shown that inflammation triggers increased production of cholesterol. The body attempts to protect the lining of blood vessels and arteries from damage, often leading to harmful levels of build-up and serious cardiovascular issues.*

Elevated CRP Levels:

High levels of CRP are an indication that inflammation is present in your body. The data linking high levels of CRP to increased heart risk has led a growing number of physicians to routinely run a test for cardiac-specific C-reactive protein.*

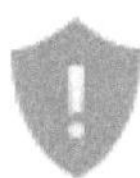 **Aches and Pains:**
Silent inflammation creates heightened pain sensitivity in the body, as well as common everyday aches and pains in joints and muscles. If your body feels sore and stiff, systematic inflammation is likely to blame.[*]

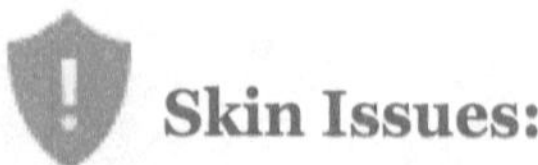 **Skin Issues:**

Silent inflammation is the hallmark of the redness, itchiness, flaky skin and discomfort associated with many common skin conditions.*

 **Digestive Discomfort:**

The gut microbiome is so complex, it is sometimes referred to as a "second brain." And while there are many factors that can disrupt its delicate balance, digestive issues can often be traced to harmful inflammation within the digestive tract.*

Chapter Two
Wellness Plan

a. A wellness plan for seniors over sixty
b.   Wellness plan is a set of actions and habits that can help you
c. maintain or improve your health and well-being as you age.
d. There is no one-size-fits-all plan, *See some general guidelines below:*

•   See your healthcare provider regularly. Even if you feel perfectly healthy, you should see your provider at least once a year for a checkup. Your provider can screen you for common health problems, such as high blood pressure, diabetes, osteoporosis, and certain cancers. They can also advise you on the best preventive measures, such as vaccinations, supplements, and medications, for your specific needs.

•   Eat a balanced and nutritious diet. In later life, you still need healthy food, but fewer calories. Aim for a variety of foods from different food groups, especially fruits, vegetables, whole grains, lean protein, and low-fat dairy. These foods can provide you with essential vitamins, minerals, antioxidants, and fiber that can protect your health and lower your risk of chronic

diseases. Avoid processed foods, added sugars, saturated fats, and trans fats as much as possible.

• Stay physically active. Physical activity can help you maintain your strength, balance, flexibility, and endurance. It can also improve your mood, cognitive function, and quality of life. The Centers for Disease Control and Prevention (CDC) recommends that older adults get at least 150 minutes of moderate-intensity aerobic activity (such as brisk walking) and two or more days of muscle-strengthening activity (such as lifting weights) per week. You can also do activities that improve your balance (such as tai chi) and flexibility (such as yoga) to prevent falls and injuries.
• Keep your mind sharp. Mental stimulation can help you prevent or delay cognitive decline and dementia. You can

challenge your brain by learning new skills, taking up hobbies, reading books, playing games, solving puzzles, or taking classes. You can also boost your brain health by staying socially connected with your family, friends, neighbors, or community groups. Social interaction can reduce stress, loneliness, and depression.

• Take care of your emotional well-being. Aging can bring many changes and challenges that can affect your mental health. You may experience loss of loved ones, retirement, isolation, chronic pain, or illness. It is normal to feel sad, anxious, or stressed at times, but if these feelings persist or interfere with your daily life, you should seek professional help.

• You can also cope with negative emotions by practicing relaxation techniques (such as deep breathing or meditation), expressing yourself through art or music, seeking support from others who understand what you are going through, or joining a support group.

• Lower your risk of falls and fractures. Falls are the leading cause of injury and death among older adults. They can cause serious injuries such as hip fractures or head trauma that can limit your mobility and independence. To prevent falls, you should make sure your home is safe and free of hazards (such as loose rugs or cords), wear sturdy shoes that fit well and have good traction, use assistive devices (such as a cane or walker) if needed, and get regular eye exams to check for vision problems. You should also take steps to keep your bones strong and healthy by getting enough calcium and vitamin D from your diet or supplements, doing weight-bearing exercises (such as walking or jogging), and avoiding smoking and excessive alcohol consumption.

- Use sunscreen daily. Sun exposure can cause skin damage, wrinkles, age spots, and skin cancer. To protect your skin from the harmful effect of the sun, you should apply sunscreen with at least SPF 15 every day before going outside. [1]. You should also wear protective clothing (such as hats, sunglasses, long sleeves) and seek shade when possible.

- Quit smoking. Smoking is one of the most preventable causes of death and disease in the world. It can damage almost every organ in your body and increase your risk of lung cancer, heart disease, stroke, chronic obstructive pulmonary disease (COPD), and many other conditions. Quitting smoking can improve your health and longevity at any age. If you need help to quit smoking, you can talk to your healthcare provider about nicotine replacement therapy (such as patches or gum), prescription medications (such as bupropion or varenicline), counseling (such as phone or online support), or other resources (such as apps or websites). These are some of the ways you can create a wellness plan for yourself if you are over sixty. Remember that everyone is different and what works for one person may not work for another. You should consult with your healthcare provider before making any major changes to your lifestyle or starting any new exercise program or diet plan. They can help you tailor a plan that suits your individual needs and goals.

Chapter Three
Promise to Myself

I promised myself when I turned Sixty-five, I would make sure that I was in good health. I wanted to be able to play with my granddaughter without getting out of breath and go on trips with my husband and work my business. my blood pressure was high my cholesterol was high my weight was unstable, and I was stressed in my Executive Position. The age of sixty-five was coming. I saw my husband was in good health in his Seventies and he was juicing to contribute to his good health. I tried some of his juice receipts. I did not like the taste of it. Yet I continued to watch him day after day looking and feeling great.

I decided that I would do research on how to take care of the whole person in my senior years. I did my research interviewed Doctors and nurses and used my experience in healthcare for over forty years as well as my years in nutrition for twenty years. Have your ever in your life knew what to do but did not do it? That was me partially following the advice I gave others professionally. Other people my age, some in good shape and some not in good shape. I began to juice, take care of my finances, work on my self-esteem, spirituality, as well as love and relationships.

I noticed that my husband was not on high blood pressure medication, he was not on cholesterol medication no diabetes wasn't even taken an aspirin and was the happiness person I knew. I looked at myself and I had high blood pressure medication and cholesterol medication and taking the aspirin. I decided to make a change to being more fabulous at Sixty-five. I began juicing. I looked at my finances relationship and personal development and I went to work

Question:

What do you want to do with the rest of your life? I worked in health care for forty years in geriatrics. There are Many people in the nursing homes who do not want to be there. Age 30,40, 50,60 and up. Have you decided what quality of life you want to live? Do you want to take trips Do you want to have energy for your grandchildren? Do you want to have stability in your finances, your love and relationships How is your self-esteem Have you done some work on your personal development? I do not know what part of the journey you are in; however, I know that we are better together. Take this journey with me and let us be the best that we can be. Pain free after sixty not only stand for pain free in your body but mind body soul and spirit. Come on, let do this.

Chapter Four
Fruits good for juicing and eating

Are you struggling with joint pain? If you are suffering from joint discomfort in your knees, wrists, or another part of your body, you are not alone. Millions of people are miserable by this pain as well. They have to pay a myriad of money to treat the pain with medications. However, through much medical research, using some pain medications in a long term has its side effects and complications.

GOOD NEWS: is that you can also relieve pain by some particular fruits. Fruits contain various vitamins and antioxidants which can help to treat inflammation that help to relieve joint pain and discomfort.

Six Fruits and how they aid in relief of pain

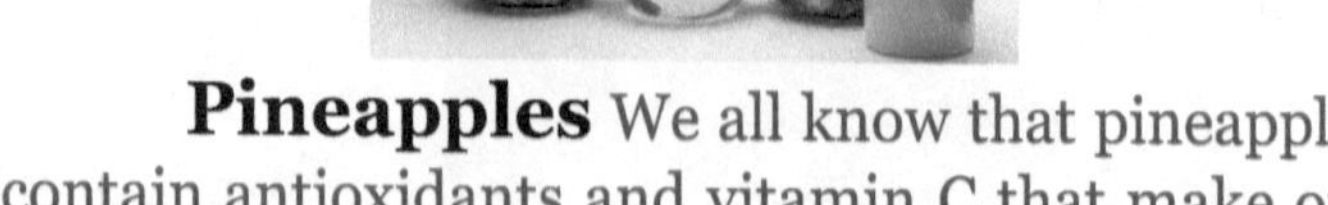

Pineapples We all know that pineapples contain antioxidants and vitamin C that make our immune system stronger and play a vitally important role in treating inflammation. But that is not all, pineapples also contributing to alleviating joint pain as well. According to scientific studies, pineapples supplies bromelain which is used to relieve pain in trauma or surgery.

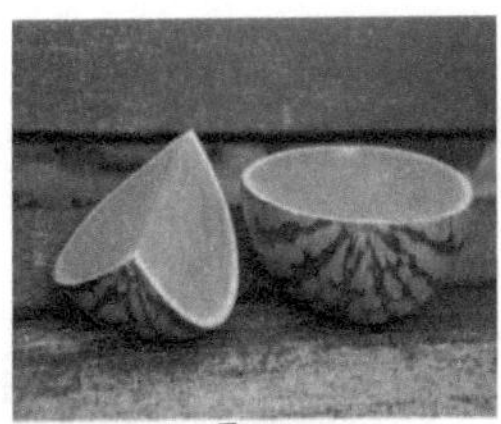

Watermelon is a great source of carotenoid beta-cryptoxanthin which lesson inflammation symptoms, therefore relieve the pain. You can squeeze watermelon to get watermelon juice, or you can also directly eat every day. Your body will thank you for its good result in reducing pain.

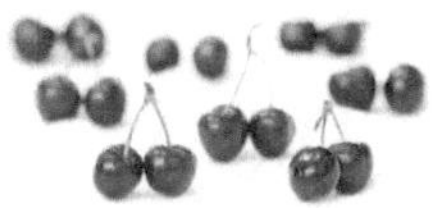

Cherries are the first thing we would highly recommend to you because cherries have a certain amount of antioxidants. Some research has shown that cherries help to dwindle the frequency of joint pain and have good results in inflammation treatment by the amount of anthocyanins found in cherries. Therefore, cherries would be a perfect home remedy for treating joint pain and inflammation. Through many scientific studies, we found that it would be ideal if you eat 10 to 12 cherries on a daily basis for 20-day period.

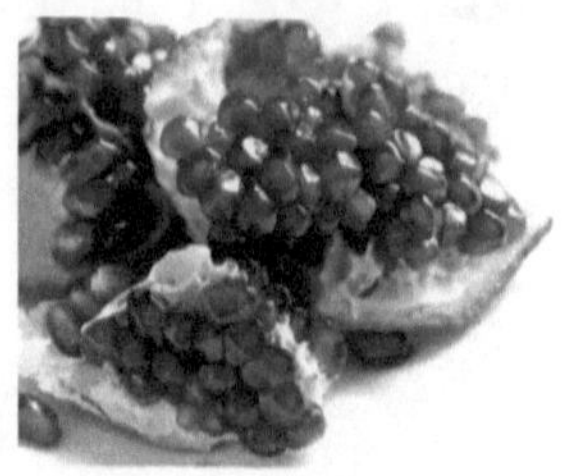

Pomegranates have a lot of nutrients that provides a variety of essential nutritious components that is beneficial to our health. In particular, it has an extremely rich source of antioxidants. You will feel much better if you add one pomegranate to your daily diet whether you eat the whole ones or drink juice. A number of researchers reported that this special fruit can also use in preventing bone damage and reduce joint pain in inflammation

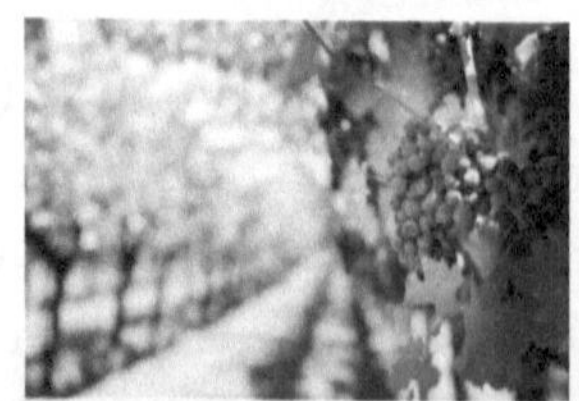

Grapes regardless of what kind of grapes- black or green, are amazing kinds of fruit we should add to our diet on a regular basis. They are not only

nutritious but also full of natural and effectively healing power. A Harvard School of Public Health study has shown that anthocyanidins found in grapes reduce inflammation and joint pain.

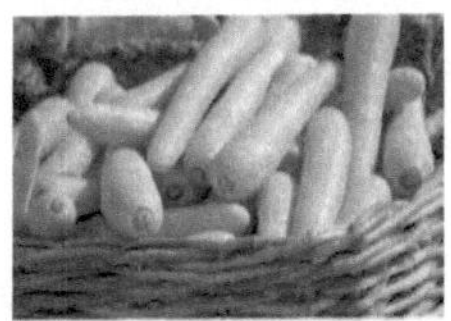

Carrots another recommendation is carrot, one of the great fruits to treat joint pain at home if you do not want to use pain relief medication. Beta-cryptoxanthin was found in carrots which are powerful antioxidants. It helps to reduce the risks for joint pain and prevent rheumatoid arthritis. As a colored fruit carrots have the properties to reduce inflammation of planar fascia as well as swelling of different parts of the body.

Now we can see how important fruit is in the aiding of being relieved of pain. Juicing or eating these fruits can make a dramatic difference to your health.

Chapter Five
Vegetables for Juicing and eating

Six vegetables and how they aid in relief of pain

Broccoli

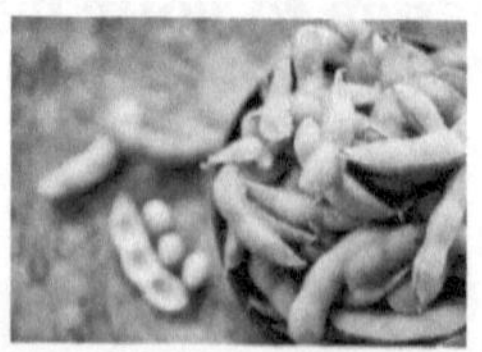

This cruciferous vegetable may be best known for cancer prevention, but did you know it might also minimize post-exercise muscle soreness? Here's why. When you work out hard, your body produces inflammatory cytokines that do a number on your muscles (hello, tired, achy muscles!). Turns out, eating broccoli after a workout could nip that process in the bud.

Edamame

Yes, these young soybeans are veggies too! "Soy is rich in isoflavones, plant compounds that may help reduce the risk of chronic inflammation-related diseases such as heart disease and diabetes," says Salge Blake. In a 2018 study published in the Journal of Diabetes & Diabetes & Metabolic Disorders. , volunteers with type 2 diabetes who ate 1 cup of cooked soybeans three times weekly for eight weeks reduced their levels of C-reactive protein (CRP), a marker of inflammation.

Mushrooms

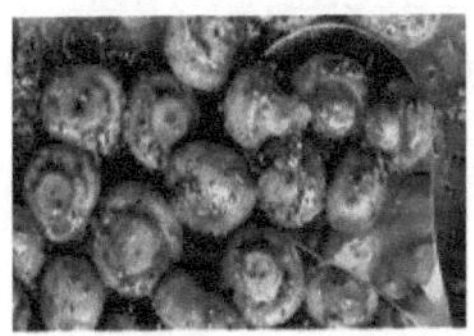

Diabetes and inflammation tend to travel together, per a 2019 article in the European Cardiology Review. But what if there was a food that could reduce diabetes-related inflammation? According to some research, that food is mushrooms. These fungi contain ergothioneine, an antioxidant that

Herbs in recipes

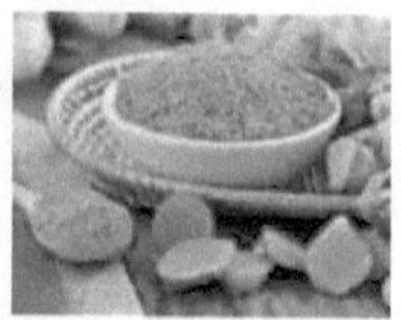

Turmeric

is a product of Curcuma longa, a rhizomatous herbaceous perennial plant belonging to the ginger family Zingiberaceae, which is a native tropical South Asia, as many as 133 species of Curcuma have been identified worldwide. Turmeric is the golden spice.

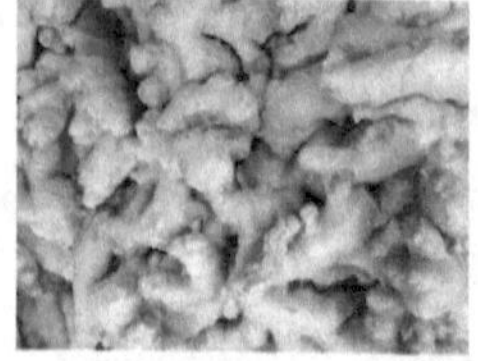

Ginger in small doses

8 health benefits of ginger and side effects.

1. Antioxidant properties

Gingerol is the main bioactive compound in ginger and has powerful anti-inflammatory and antioxidant properties. For example, it can help with decreasing oxidative stress and minimizing free radical damage in the body.

2. Eases nausea

Ginger has been found to be effective against nausea and may help with easing nausea and vomiting for people who need to undergo specific surgeries. Ginger may likewise help chemotherapy-related nausea. Pregnant women can use ginger to alleviate pregnancy -related nausea, such as morning sickness.

3. Fights germs

Certain chemical compounds in ginger help the body fight off germs and are particularly good at stopping the growth of microorganisms, such as E coli and Shigella. They can also keep viruses such as respiratory syncytial virus under control.

4. Soothes sore muscles

Ginger will not relieve muscle pain immediately, but it may ease soreness over the long run. Some studies have shown that people with muscle pain who took ginger regularly had less pain the next day than the people who did not.

5. Eases arthritis symptoms

Because ginger has anti-inflammatory properties, it can be particularly useful for treating symptoms of both rheumatoid arthritis and osteoarthritis.

6. Helps manage blood sugar

Ginger can help the body use insulin better. However, more research is required to confirm whether ginger can help improve glucose levels.

7. Helps lower cholesterol levels

Eating ginger every day may help lower "bad" or low-density lipoprotein (LDL) Cholesterol levels in the body. In one study, taking 5 grams of ginger a day for almost 5 months was linked with lowering LDL Cholesterol an average of 30 points.

8. Aids in weight loss

Gingerols and shogaols can help improve the body's metabolic rate and thus help with weight loss.

Can you eat too much ginger?

Side effects from eating ginger are rare, but the following can occur if you eat too much:

- Heartburn
- Gas
- Stomachache
- Burning sensation in the mouth

Avoid taking ginger when on any kind of medication because it can interact negatively and cause discomfort. May increase levels of an anti-inflammatory hormone that people with type 2 diabetes often don't produce enough of called adiponectin

Carrots

Munching on carrots does more than help keep your eyes healthy. These root vegetables may also stomp out inflammation, one of the primary mechanisms behind colon cancer. A 2020 Nutrients study that tracked 57,053 volunteers for 18 years found that people who reported eating two to four raw carrots a week were 17% less likely to develop colon cancer than those who never ate raw carrots

The Bottom Line

Eating plenty of colorful veggies and fruits is one of the best ways to put the brakes on chronic inflammation

Chapter Six
Four: Juicing Recipes- Cold Drinks

Help with Pain and inflammation

Ground turmeric – fresh root

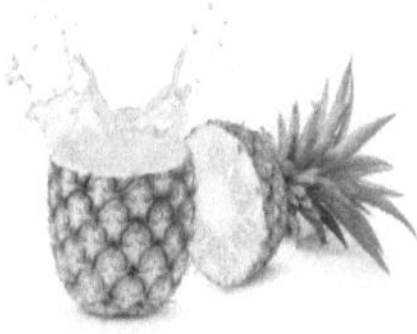

Peel turmeric and ginger
- Frozen pineapple chunks
- Banana blend until smooth
- Strain
- Drink

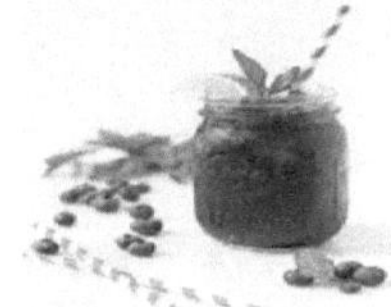

Blueberry blend
- Blueberries
- Coconut water
- Frozen Banana
- 1 Tablespoon flaxseed
- Drink and enjoy

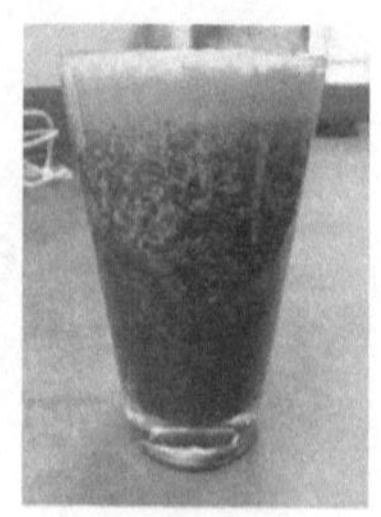

Green Juice Anti-inflammatory

- Lime juice fresh
- Apple
- Cucumber
- Kale
- Cucumber
- Celery
- Add cucumber and apple first to blender
- Blend and strain

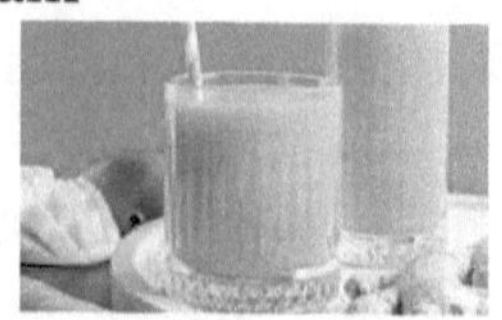

Anti-inflammatory Carrot Juice

- Carrots
- Beets medium
- Apple
- Orange
- 1 cup water
- Ginger

Lorraine Anti-inflammatory coffee

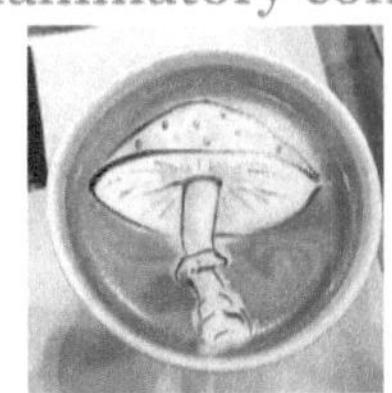

A morning shot
Mushroom Coffee

Shake ground turmeric in coffee drink as
usual

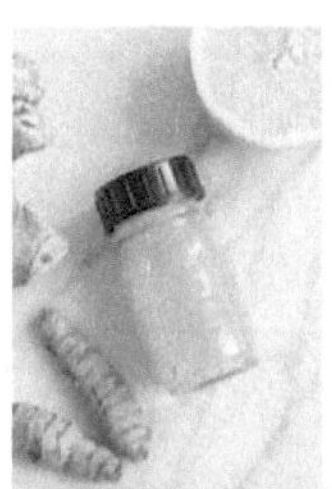

Ginger Shot anti-inflammatory

- ¼ cup chopped Ginger
- ¼ cup Coconut water
- Chayenne pepper-
- Boil- strain
- Lemon slice
- Drink at once Note: spicy

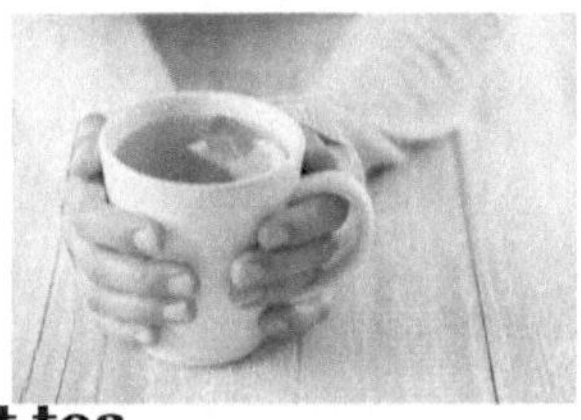

Lorraine -Hot tea
for sleep and relief of pain

- Juice for pain
- Pineapple skins
- Lemon peel
- Lime peel
- Cinnamon
- Honey
- Turmeric peel
- Ginger peel
- Bring to boil – let sit for 2 hours-drink as needed.

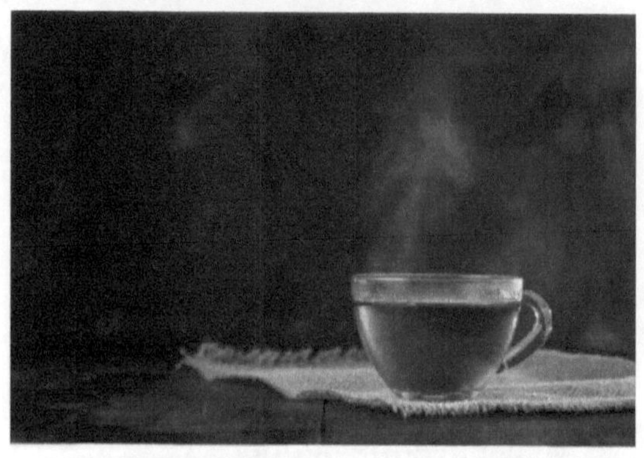

Anti-inflammatory hot tea

- 2 cups water
- Ground turmeric
- Black pepper
- Honey strain
- Simmer ten minutes

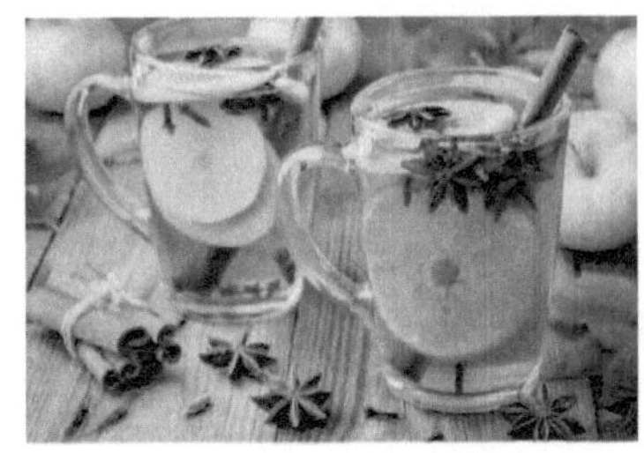

Donnie Ray weight loss tea
Drink hot or cold

cup Water
¼ cup Blueberries
½ Banana
¼ strawberries
Sprinkle Cinnamon
Cup spinach
¼ Beet root

Wrapping Up Part One of Our Series on Living Pain-Free

Thank you for joining me on this journey to a pain-free life. If you've been taking notes, I hope you've found this information helpful and are ready to make a change in your health. Congratulations on taking the first step!

It's important to remember that this is not a quick fix. I've noticed that when I maintain a healthy diet and drink plenty of fluids, I feel significantly better. However, if I stray from this plan for over a week, my pain returns. So, don't get discouraged if you don't see immediate results! Be consistent and keep moving forward, and you will eventually start seeing positive changes.

Together, let's strive towards a better quality of life. We all deserve to live well, regardless of our age. Join me on social media for discussions and tips on living pain-free, especially after the age of sixty.

My Notes to be pain free

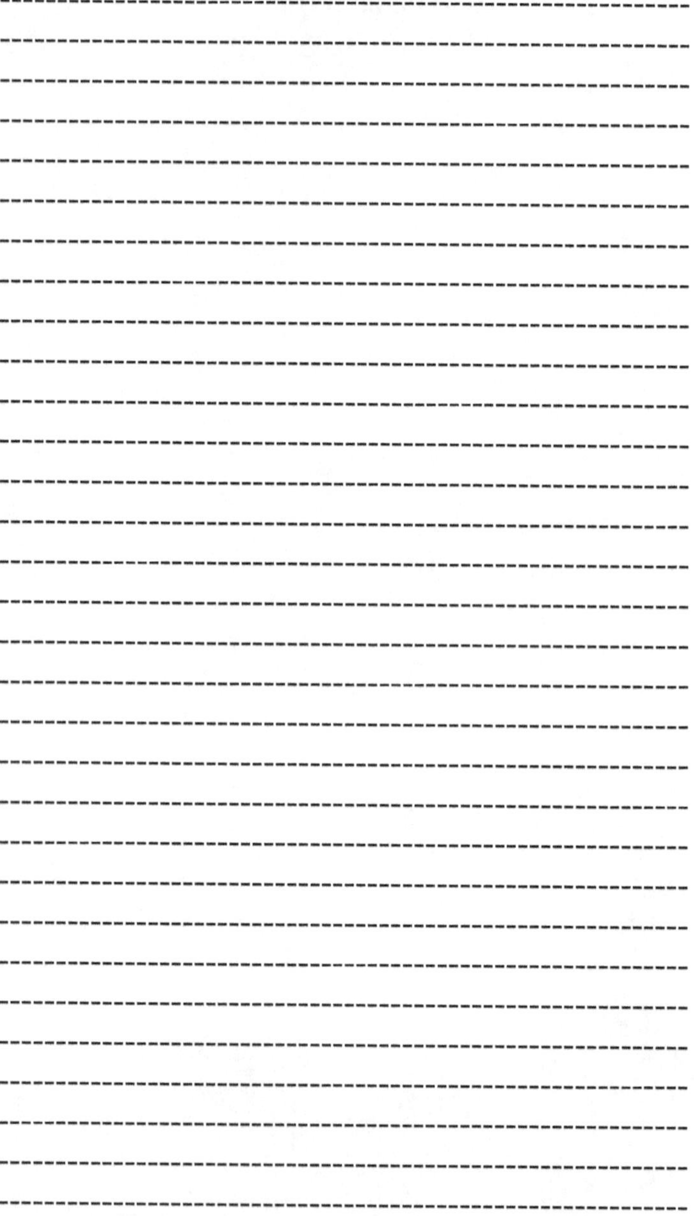

Meet the Author

Lorraine Jenkins-Wilkes,

the Storytellers Coach and CEO of The   Write Path Publishing Consultants LLC. Is a Multi -International Best Selling-Author. Lorraine's company works with business owners, ministers, content creators, and professionals from all over the world. She has created over 10,000 diet plans for the geriatric community and is a Certified Life Recovery Coach, Certified Master Storyteller, and an Ordained Minister. The Host and Visionary of The Power of S.H.E. Radio show and Social Media Ministry, Lorraine has earned a bachelor's degree in Theology, as well as a Degree in Nutrition and Administration.

Her most cherished treasures are her marriage, three adult children, and granddaughter. Lorraine is a firm believer in the healing power of laughter and good living.

Her career as a Corporate Executive in the Healthcare field spanned over 40 years. After experiencing chronic pain and seeing several doctors with no solution, Lorraine

Decided to take her health into her own hands. With the help of holistic methods to decrease pharmaceuticals, she not only found relief but discovered that she could help others too.

Booking Information

For keynote speaking engagements

The Write Path Publishing consultants LLC

Website www.twppublishing.com

Email writingcoachlorraine@gmail.com

Disclaimer

These claims have not been evaluated by the food and drug administration The information in this book is for educational or informational purposes only and should not be considered a substitute for professional medical advice or consultation with healthcare professionals. Please consult your doctor for medical information before starting or using any of the recipes in this book. This book offers useful tips that I have used to maintain my health.

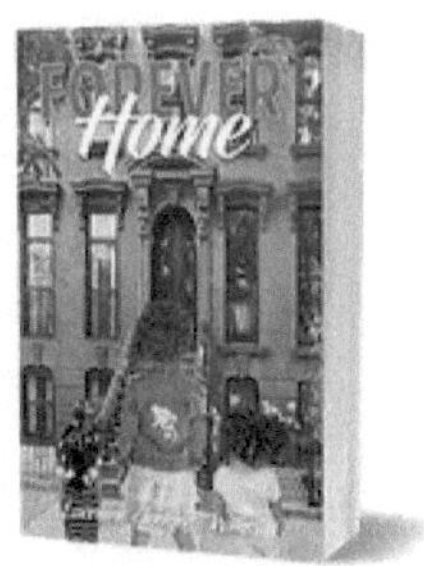

Lorraine's Publishing's

- Forever Home
- Courage to Change
- Courage to change Devotional
- First Ladies Voice
- Power of S.H.E. Devotional
- The Guide for a new Pastor Wife
- Rising with the Son (Collaboration)
- How to Publish your eBook in 30 days
- Rising with the Son Look what the Lord has done (Collaboration)
- How to Survive a Toxic Leader - Collaboration
- Amazon.com

www.ingramcontent.com/pod-product-compliance
Lightning Source LLC
Chambersburg PA
CBHW021139260726
48656CB00023B/972